The Science
and Theology
of Essential Oils
a study guide

Dr. Marcus O. Durham, PhD, ThD

Dream Point Publishers

⇐ ⇑ ⇒

The Science and Theology of Essential Oils
a study guide

Author: Marcus O. Durham, PhD, ThD
Cover photo: courtesy Rosemary Durham, goat's rue on hillside at our ranch.
Printed in United States of America

First printing, July 15, 2016
Edition: 160725

ISBN: 978-1535244985

THEWAY LABS
Laboratories / Failure Analysis / Energy Consultants
Electrical, Petro-chemical, Natural
www.ThewayLabs.com

17350 E US 64 Hwy
Bixby, OK 74008
918-496-8709

Our friends in the study group, who asked me to do a series on essential oils.
You have contributed to my knowledge base.
You have been a joy to let me hold forth.

The purpose of life is to be all you can be.

Table of Contents

THE SCIENCE AND THEOLOGY OF ESSENTIAL OILS

Dr. Marcus O. Durham, PhD, ThD

Deus in singulis est: God is in the detail.

Let your food be your medicine, and your medicine be your food: Hippocrates

There is no magic, no oouh-oouh spirits, and no wizardry to essential oils. It is just science: Dr MOD

PREFACE

A note about the format of the paragraphs is in order.
The single sentence format provides an easier outline for use in classes, seminars, and discussions.
The structure of the information aids reference, rather than simply reading as a novel.

When discussing essential oils, representative samples are highly recommended for sensory association.
Note, aroma bypasses the logical brain and goes straight to the limbic or emotional center.
The material is an effective 8-hour seminar.

BACKGROUND

The Nobel Prize in chemistry was awarded for essential oil research to Professor Otto Wallach in 1910.
Essential oils are not new and are very real, even if society does not understand.
But then again society seldom understands science.
If one does not understand, he tends to dismiss the science behind the technology.
> *What we do not understand, we dismiss or think is magic.*---MOD

Essential is the word essence, which simply means aromatic.
Perhaps 'essencial' would be a better pronunciation, even if not proper English.
Plants make non-aromatic fatty oils (aliphatic, chain) and fragrant essential oils (alicyclic, ring).
Mineral oils, called hydrocarbons, have a similar composition.
The other source of oil is in animal fat.

The smell and flavor of herbs and flowers is the essential oils in the plant and dried parts.
Another form of oil is the oleo-gum-resin, which is simply the sap.
Resin is extracted in different ways, including crushing and draining, depending on the species.

Aromatic oil consists of tiny molecules of less than 500 atomic mass units (amu).
Non-aromatic oils are much larger, up to 1000 amu.
The extremely small molecules can migrate across cells.

One (1) drop of essential oil has over 4e19 molecules.
That is 4, with 19 zeroes after it.
One drop can cover every body cell with 400,000 molecules.
Obviously, using only a tiny amount of oil is necessary to obtain the benefit.

Aromatic, essential oils are widely used in very diverse ways, including:
disinfectant, solvent, cleanser, perfume, flavoring, medicine (physical), emotional, and spiritual.

Of the five senses – see, hear, touch, taste, and smell- four senses go through the logical brain.
Smell goes directly to limbic system, which is the seat of emotions.
The limbic includes thalmus, hypothalmus, corpus callosum, fornix, pineal, and pituitary glands.
The neural cortex and endocrine glands are responsible for hormones.
> *We do not know what we do not know.* ---old adage

BIBLE BASIS

The Bible mentions 33 species of aromatic plants and over 180 references to plants and their oils.
Some authors report a much larger number by including a mixture as a reference to all the components.
Culture and history shows many other plants and oils were also enjoyed at the time of writing.
The very first chapter affirms plants were for use by people.

As has been noted, this first chapter is amazing since validation of the sequence occurred in the 1990's.
Interestingly, the writer inscribed the record about 1500 BCE, 3500 years before contemporary science.
How could the writer have possibly known the big bang explanation and progression at that time?

> *And God said, Let the earth bring forth grass, the herb yielding seed, and the fruit tree yielding fruit after his kind, whose seed is in itself, upon the earth: and it was so. And the earth brought forth grass, and herb yielding seed after his kind, and the tree yielding fruit, whose seed was in itself, after his kind: and God saw that it was good.*
> --Genesis 1:11-12 KJV

> *Then God said, "I now give you every seed-bearing plant on the face of the entire earth and every tree that has fruit with seed in it. They will be yours for food."*
> --Genesis 1:29 NET

The first specific discussion of essential oils is the history of Joseph's indenture to Arab traders.

> *Then they sat down to eat a meal. They looked up, and there was a caravan of Ishmaelites coming from Gilead. Their camels were carrying aromatic gum, balsam, and resin, going down to Egypt.*
> --Genesis 37:25 HCSB

Genesis states the merchants were carrying spices, balm, and resin about 1700 BCE.
Note herbs' active ingredients are oils.
Our ground spices had not come into common use in ancient times.

Consider the event was the first individual of the Jewish people, who migrated to Egypt.
The exodus occurred some 250 years later, when Moses gave the Law and rules for tabernacle worship.
Clearly, the use of essential oils predated the law and ceremony.

Common religious practice refers to uncomprehended events as spiritual or ceremonial.
Unskilled and even some translations refer to herbs, spices, and oils as ceremonial, like food laws.
A few translations even erroneously insert olive before the word oil, when essential oils are involved.
We know the food laws and practices had a rational basis to promote health and mitigate spread of disease.

The act of eating clean food predated the flood, so it was not a legal or ceremonial practice.
Genesis 7 affirms that two of every animal and 7 of clean animals were selected for protection.
Similarly, there were real reasons for use of aromatics during those ancient times.
Consider the very first recorded residence was among the fragrance of the garden at Eden.

Note that in translation, not all authorities agree.
Because of the ancient language, the exact contemporary name may be in question.
Regardless, the evidence is overwhelming that oils, herbs, and plant parts existed for cleaning, food, medicine, and perfume.
The process of steam-distilled oils currently enjoyed was likely unknown in biblical times.
The oils, resins, and spices employed would be in a different form.
Since some aromatics were in resin form rather than liquid, heated incense diffused the molecules.
Nevertheless, the process of determining the usage can be instructive.

BIBLE LIST

The following names the significant essential oils compiled from the Ancient record.
The list illustrates the complexity of oils employed thousands of years ago which are still invoked.
Some of these are common, but others have limited availability as oils, but are available as spices.
In later sections, the history, chemistry, and application of these aromatics are limned.

> Acacia/shittah/gum arabic (acacia Arabica/farnesiana)
> Aloes/sandalwood (santalum album)
> Anise (pimpenella anisum)
> Bay (laurilus nobilis)
> Balm / balsam (commiphora erythraea/opobalsamum)
> Calamus/cane (acorus calamus)
> Cassia (cinnamomum cassia)
> Cedarwood (cedrus atlantica)
> Cinnamon (cinnamomum verum)
> Cistus /labdanum/ rose of Sharon (cistus ladanifer)
> Coriander (coriandrum sativum)
> Cumin (cuminum cyminum)
> Cypress (cupressus sempervirens)
> Dill (anethum graveolens)
> Fir (abies alba)
> Frankincense (olibanum -- boswellia carteri)

Galbanum (ferula gummosa)
Henna (lawsonia inermis)
Hyssop (hyssopus officinalis)
Juniper (juniperus osteosperma)
Mint (mentha longifolia)
Myrrh /stacte (commiphora myrrha)
Myrtle (myrtus communis)
Narcissus / rose of Isaiah (narcissus tazetta)
Onycha (styrax benzoin)
Pine (pinus sylvestris)
Rue (ruta graveolens)
Saffron (crocus sativus)
Spikenard (nardostachys jatamansi)
Terebinth / pistachio (pistacia terebinthus)
Wormwood / absinthe /bitters (artemesia judiaca)

Bdellium /African myrrh (commiphora africana) is similar to common myrrh, but produces less oil

Mustard (brassica nigra) is used as a spice and flavoring, but avoided as oil. Mustard contains > 92% allyl isothiocyanate otherwise known as the basis of mustard gas and similar to cyanide.

TRADITION, TRADITION

Essential oils provided chemical benefits many thousands of years ago.
Why are they not more common today?
Oils, spices, and herbs were routine medicine until WWII, when drugs began replacing them.
Work by Leopold Ruzieka and others showed chemistry could make synthetic constituents for the oils.

A significant problem arises from created synthetics.
The synthetics may have the same mass structure, but do not have same electric-magnetic and frequency profile, as seen in the unified energy equation discussed in the physics section.
Consequently, the synthetics do not precisely match the receptors in the biological system.
Lacking the appropriate electric-magnetic frequency profile, the synthetics cannot resonate.
Chemical interaction with receptors may behave as stimulating, blocking, or blocking complimentary compounds.

The synthetics become drugs.
The advantage of synthetics is every production is pure and exactly the same in each process.
The disadvantage is modification of the natural substance, which is necessary to obtain patents.
But, the patent is necessary to sell drugs at substantial cost and to require a prescription.

Because of the inability to match biological receptors, side effects are often worse than benefits.
Issues that are even more serious arise from mixing drugs due to counter interaction between the drugs.
An important caution is synthetic drugs do not cure; they are used to treat symptoms.

Dr. Robert S. Mendelsohn, MD, describes the allopathic religion in *Confessions of a Medical Heretic.*
People regard medicine with more faith than a religion.

Doctors are revered as priests.
Hospitals are the temple.
Medical miracles come from dispensing holy waters (drugs, serums, antibiotics).
The industry performs rituals and sacrifices (radiation and surgery).
The loyal tithe to medical insurance through coercion .

What is the consequence of this newfound religious fervor?
Adverse drug reactions cause admission of two (2) million people per year.
Over 100,000 per year die from 'proper' drug administration.
The Journal of American Medical Association (JAMA) reports over 250,000 deaths / year from doctor treatment.

Compare those staggering statistics to reports from American Association of Poison Control Centers.
Plant caused illness had 2 fatalities and 53 serious poisonings.
The plants were not medicinal but common houseplants and shrubs.
Statistics show 30 fatalities per year from weight loss mixes, which are quasi medicinal.
Available published documents show NO serious or fatal poisonings as a result from essential oils.
Nevertheless, be aware.

Compare the medicinal effect of just one essential oil to antibiotics.
Prescribed antibiotics kill bacteria, which necessarily includes many biotics, even friendly gut bacteria.
Antibiotics create resistant strains, when every attacked bacteria is not destroyed.
Since the drugs are very specific pure design, a few bacteria escape who are not responsive.
MRSA (methicillin-resistant staphylococcus aureus) and E coli are resistant strains found in hospitals.

Oil of Onycha (styrax benzoin) dissolved in alcohol (called Tincture of Benzoin) was hospitals' most effective antiseptic and antibacterial agent.
The tincture even destroyed resistant strains, but the common oil compound is not patentable.
A cinnamon oil solution is as effective as the antibiotics penicillin and ampicillin.
Antibiotics are effective only against bacteria, not viruses or other microbes.
In contrast, essential oils are broad spectrum, with many being anti-microbial.

Oils are very concentrated and strong, which may cause allergic reactions, particularly skin irritation.
Some essential oils are biocides, which effectively kill all microorganisms.
So, in concentration they are potentially deleterious.
Use only a small amount.
Do not apply many oils in neat form.
Place only a few drops in a carrier oil to dilute.

If a reaction occurs, avoid water.
Rather apply a carrier oil to further dilute the effect.
Since some oils are used for food flavoring, obviously those oils can be ingested if food grade.

> *"Never must the physician say, the disease is incurable. By that admission he denies God,*
> *our Creator; he doubts Nature with her profuseness of hidden powers and mysteries."*
> --Morris Fishbein, M.D. , editor of JAMA, from his book *THE MEDICAL FOLLIES*, 1925

That is an interesting quote by Fishbein for numerous reasons.

The title of his book gives the clue.

Although an MD, he apparently did not practice medicine with patients.

As the 'authoritative' mouthpiece of the AMA for many years, he likely did more in an attempt to discredit natural healing and alternative medicine than any other individual did in the last century.

Furthermore, he was largely responsible for removing nutrition from medical training.

To him, anyone outside his narrow perception was a quack, who he proceeded to destroy.

Unfortunately, vestiges of his intolerant lack of knowledge continue to perpetuate in society.

Now who is the quack?

The medical profession has developed a fantastic diagnostic system and treatment for acute conditions.

However, chronic care has been somewhat less effective.

Symptomatic care appears to be the norm.

Use allopathic where appropriate, but be aware that tradition has a reason.

SOME SIGNIFICANT WORDS

Three Hebrew words and a Greek biblical word provide insight in the context of oils.

Remember, the Hebrew writing came about 3500 years ago.

The Greek writing was over 2,000 years ago.

The translation into Old English was over 400 years ago.

Therefore, the religious words will likely have a more contemporary meaning than the translation.

Also note, the early Hebrew was written without vowel pointing, so only the consonants are shown.

A comparison of the traditional English, the exotic, then the contemporary English shows the transition.

Anoint: Hebrew is *m-s-ch*, which simply means 'rub'.

Apothecary or perfumer: Hebrew is *r-q-ch*, which simply means 'mix or compound'.

Incense: Hebrew is *q-t-r-th*, which simply means aromatic resin or spice

Sorcerer or witchcraft: Greek is *pharmakeia*, which simply means pharmacy.

Consider the context of the traditional English word anoint.

The Hebrew may be pronounced 'masach', which is similar to our 'massage'.

The meaning is 'rub'.

The term ointment is from the same root.

The similarity should not be surprising, since English anoint and ointment are also the same root.

Ointment derives its odor from essential oils or components.

The Hebrew is the same root as Messiah.

The Greek translation is Christos, which also simply means anointed.

Great beauty and intrigue explodes with a little research and understanding of history.

HEALING APPLICATIONS

One of the intriguing applications of essential oils is medicinal, in times of yore.

Three different types of healing transpired, as identified by the Greek notations.

Iaomai denotes 'instant', which some regard as miraculous.

Therapeuo defines 'therapy or take care of', which is a progressive process.
Sozo describes the complete 'body, soul, and spirit' otherwise called physical, emotional, and mental.

Mark 5:25-34 shares the report of a woman who spent all her money on physicians.
But, no one could cure her.
She came to see the Rabbi, where she was totally, instantly healed.

Jesus did not claim to heal; he said 'your faith has made you whole.'
His acts were not random or placed on everyone he saw.
He only helped people who came to him or requested aid.

Three references provide key elements relevant to aid and assistance to those in need.

> *And he said unto her, Daughter, thy faith hath made thee whole; go in peace, and be whole of thy plague.*
> --Mark 5:34 KJV

What is the first application?

A positive attitude is necessary on the part of the receiver.

> *Is anyone among you sick? Then he must call for the elders of the church and they are to pray over him, anointing him with oil in the name of the Lord;*
> --James 5:14

What is the second application?

Medicinal oil is necessary.
Like priests, the elders were assumed knowledgeable in essential medicinal oils.

> *Calling the Twelve to him, he began to send them out two by two and gave them authority over impure spirits.*
> *These were his instructions: "Take nothing for the journey except a staff—no bread, no bag, no money in your belts. Wear sandals but not an extra shirt.*
> *Whenever you enter a house, stay there until you leave that town. And if any place will not welcome you or listen to you, leave that place and shake the dust off your feet as a testimony against them."*
> *They went out and preached that people should repent. They drove out many demons and anointed many sick people with oil and healed them.*
> --Mark 6:7-13 NIV

What are three other applications?

1. Do not waste time with people, who do not believe or accept the treatment.
   Do not even think about them. They choose if they want help.
2. Healing comes after change from what you have been doing. Repent means change.
3. Healing involves things not readily apparent, which includes body, soul, and spirit.

What are demons, if not negative spirits?
We are well aware of influences, which are not physically apparent.
Resonance with these influences is a mental choice.

NOW, JUST A LITTLE CHEMISTRY

An old query asks, "Why did God make fat?" The response is "To give food flavor."
The witticism is precisely correct. Fat is a source of flavor.
The energy in food derives from carbohydrates, proteins and fats otherwise known as lipids and oils.

Essential aromatic oils are an elegant recipe of sophisticated chemicals.
One cannot determine the flavor of a cake from the flour, oil, and liquid ingredients.
The recipe is critical.
Similarly, we cannot determine the efficacy of oils from their chemical components.
Nevertheless, the chemistry gives clues to the oil characteristics.
Synergy exists from the recipe of chemicals. The whole is greater than the sum of the parts.

An introduction to chemistry terms is beneficial.
Essential oils are organic, which mean they are carbon (C) based.
They are a hydrocarbon, which denotes hydrogen is included.
All oils, whether from plant, mineral, or animal are hydrocarbons.

Carbon with oxygen is a carbonyl molecule.
Hydrogen with oxygen is a hydroxyl molecule.

With the introduction, consider why different oils are beneficial or not.

SATURATED? OILS

The discussion of saturated and unsaturated oils weighs large in common nutrition discussions.
But, what do the terms mean?

The advice from many conventional sources is simply wrong or worse an attempt to promote a product.
In the next few sentences, you will be able to separate the myths from fact.

Oils, lipids, or fats come from three sources – plants, minerals or petroleum, and animals.
Essential oils are plant based.
Synthetic oil components are from minerals.

The simplest oils (fats) are an unbranched linear chain of carbons with hydrogen (hydrocarbons, CH_2).
Think of a string of carbons connected together with hydrogen at every perpendicular or 90^0 location.

$$H-\underset{\underset{H}{|}}{\overset{\overset{H}{|}}{C}}-\underset{\underset{H}{|}}{\overset{\overset{H}{|}}{C}}-\underset{\underset{H}{|}}{\overset{\overset{H}{|}}{C}}-\underset{\underset{H}{|}}{\overset{\overset{H}{|}}{C}}-\underset{\underset{H}{|}}{\overset{\overset{H}{|}}{C}}-\underset{\underset{H}{|}}{\overset{\overset{H}{|}}{C}}-H$$

Saturated oils mean the maximum number of hydrogens bond to the carbons.

The oils are solid at room temperature and have a higher melting temperature.
An example is coconut oil.

Monounsaturated oils have a single hydrogen missing from the chain.
They are liquid at room temperature and solid when refrigerated.
Examples are olive and avocado oils.

Unsaturated (polyunsaturated) oils have multiple empty hydrogen spaces in the string.
The empty hydrogen spaces allow other chemicals to invade the oil.
The oils are liquid.
Examples are vegetable oils like corn, sunflower, and safflower.

Seed oils like cottonseed, flax (linseed), canola (rapeseed), and soy are toxic unless fermented or highly processed.
Paint manufacture used these oils, until latex paint replaced oil-based paints.

Oxygen is one of the chemicals, which connects to the unsaturated string filling in the voids.
As we know, oxygen makes fire burn and causes rust.
Oxygenation simply means corrosion.
Oxygenation makes oils rancid.
In living beings, excessive oxygen radicals deteriorate biological cells and promote disease (corrosion).

Antioxidants retard the degeneration process.
Numerous chemicals in essential oils have anti-oxidant properties.
Essential oils have greater anti-oxidant ability than fruits, with few exceptions.

The effectiveness of an anti-oxidant is measured in the lab using an 'orac' score.
A high orac number means a much better anti-oxidant.
In case you care, orac means oxygen radical absorbance capacity

Hydrogenation is the process of adding hydrogen into the unsaturated oil chain.
Partial hydrogenation is still unsaturated, which leaves voids in the chain.
Hydrogenated is chemically modified oil without the electrical-magnetic frequency profile of natural oil.

The loss of each hydrogen atom creates a double bond between carbon atoms.
The modified bond of unsaturated oil rotates when heated.
The result converts the normal cis-fats to unhealthy trans-fats.
Trans-fats rapidly oxidize and contribute to disease.

Oil heated to its smoke point, initiates the trans-fat chemical reaction.
Every time oil is heated, the smoke point lowers more.
Coconut is predominantly saturated oil, so its smoke point is very high.
Olive is mono-saturated, so its temperature should be below 350F, depending on the grade.
Keep other unsaturated vegetable oils well below 300F, with some below 200F.
Avoid heating nut oils.
Peanut is not a true nut, has a high temperature rating, but is unsaturated.

Cooking at very high temperature requires animal fats.

The source of the fat should be from livestock eating natural food, instead of grain fed.
Grain feeding raises the omega-6 content of the fat to the level of the grain food.

The arrangement at the end of the hydrocarbon chain is the omega complex.
Saturated oils have all hydrogen bonds filled, so saturated oils do not have an omega complex.
Monounsaturated oils are predominantly omega-9 fatty acids.
Limited saturation oils include omega-7 fatty acids. Examples are buckthorn and macadamia nuts.
Polyunsaturated oils are omega-6 dominant.
Only a few plant oils have significant omega-3, in the form of ALA (alpha linolenic acid).
Examples of seeds with significant omega-3 include flax, chia, hemp, and walnuts.
Cold-water fish is the source of most omega-3 oil.

The ideal ratio of omega-3 to omega-6 in our diet is 1:1.
The typical Western diet using unsaturated fats is closer to 1:20, which is way too much omega-6.
Excessive omega-6 deteriorates biological cells and promotes disease (corrosion).

Above, we noted the simplest oils were linear chains.
Aromatic or essential oils consist of the carbons connected together so the chain forms a ring.
The ring property makes the oils volatile, meaning the molecules evaporate to form a gas.
The gas is what the nose smells.

The understanding of all the oils and their impact really is that simple.
Granted, the analysis flies in the face of advertising to sell highly processed vegetable oils as healthy.
Consider, the investigation is a simple scientific analysis with nothing to sell.

Which oil should you use for cooking? Why?
Which oil should you use for salad dressing? Why?
Which oils should you avoid altogether? Why?

Only For Nerds

The chemical formula for saturated oils (fats, hydrocarbons) is C_nH_{2n+2}.
Replacing any hydrogen with another radical creates a new chemical and characteristics.

CARRIER OILS

Plants make non-aromatic fatty oils (aliphatic, chain) and fragrant essential oils (alicyclic, ring).

Essential oils are so concentrated that only a very few drops are required to be effective.
Other less aromatic oils serve as carriers to dilute the essential oil.

The carrier allows the drop to be dispersed effectively.

The most common carrier oil is coconut.
Olive is another effective carrier.
Almond, walnut, flaxseed, and numerous lesser-known oils arise in various formulations.
However, being unsaturated makes these seed and nut oils less than acceptable to the purist.
The section on saturated oil showed the reasons for saturated preference..

Coconut oil use is primarily for cooking, as well as a carrier.
Because of its saturated characteristics, coconut heat can be hotter than most oils without changing.
By far, olive is the most used oil including uncooked food purposes.
Olive has numerous health benefits above other plant food oils.

Whether used as a food-oil or as a carrier-oil, very specific oil processing is necessary.
First, the source must be organic to reduce risk of foreign toxins.
Natural means nothing.
Virgin means the oil is the first cold press extract from the fruit.
The oil is unrefined, no chemicals are added, and the temperature is kept cool below damage point.
Extra virgin is the oil drained in the very first hour.
Unfortunately, the terms are legally undefined in the US, so cautious skepticism is necessary.
The Biblical translation of virgin oil was words such as first, beaten, or fine oil.

The second pressing applies greater pressure to obtain less quality oil.
The product designation is second, pressed, or pure.
Refined refers to oils which have been heated to drive off all aromatics.
Light or mild is second pressed oil with virgin added to enhance the flavor.

Grasping all the terms is unnecessary.
One guideline is applicable.
Organic, extra-virgin oil should be the preferred choice.

A LITTLE PMS

The ingredients of essential oils are elegant combinations of just a few component categories.
Key characteristics of the components determine the use of a particular essential oil.
Perhaps the most significant components are the PMS – phenols, monoterpenes, and sequiterpenes.

Terpenes make essential oils unique in the plant world.
Many oils have terpenes, which describes the connection of 5 carbon and 8 hydrogen atoms (C_5H_8).
Monoterpenes and sesquiterpenes have two and three of these molecule combinations respectively.

The major terpenes are limonene from citrus and pinene from conifers.
As well as being biological solvents, terpenes are industrial solvents we use to clean oil wells.

Not surprisingly, the study of chemistry of essential oils is the same as that for petroleum or mineral oils.

MAJOR COMPONENTS, HOW CONSTRUCTED, HOW USED

Grasp the next brief discussion as a cursory overview of the recipe for oils.
Memorization is not required any more than realizing that flour in a cake is ground grain, such as wheat.
If available, apply a dilute drop of cedarwood to the right thumb as a memory aid.

Being aware of the essential oil chemistry helps to explain why particular oils exist in worship as well as personal fragrances, disinfectants, and heath vehicles.

Phenols are a benzene ring + OH molecule.
The compounds are highly antioxidant.
The phenols exhibit great antiseptic, antibacterial, and disinfectant ability.
They stimulate the nervous and immune systems.
The chemical alone is skin toxic.
Large, isolated quantities may damage the liver.
Phenols are the active ingredient of Lysol®.
The chemicals clean biological receptor sites.
Oils with high content are clove, wintergreen, and melaleuca.

Sesquiterpenes are extremely small molecules.
The molecules travel across the blood-brain barrier delivering oxygen.
The sesquiterpenes exhibit anti-inflammatory and anti-allergy properties.
They are viscous and consequently less volatile.
The lower volatility makes them excellent fixatives to perpetuate the effect of other oils.
The solvent erases miswritten dna codes.
Oils with high content are sandalwood, cedarwood, myrrh, and chamomile.

Monoterpenes are extremely small molecules.
The monoterpenes exhibit anti-inflammatory, antiseptic, antiviral, and antibacterial ability.
The chemicals inhibit the accumulation of toxins.
The chemical enhances the effect of other oils making them a balancing component.
The solvent restores cell memory dna.
Oils with high content include the citrus family and conifers.

The PMS chemicals are independent hydrocarbon molecules.
The molecules may also combine with the following chemicals.
Blends of these chemicals are the predominant remaining factors in essential oils.

Alcohols are an organic derivative of water.
Alcohols are mild with little skin irritation or toxicity.
Alcohols can be oxidized (oxygen added) to change to aldehydes, ketones, and acids.
Alcohols are an ingredient for sweeteners, perfumes, fuels, and narcotics.
Alcohols resist oxidation, ie deterioration.
Consequently, alcohols have the demonstrated ability to return cells to normal functioning.
The ability is crucial to mitigate for errant cancers.
Oils with high content are rose, geranium, juniper, and tea tree.

Esters are formed from alcohol and inorganic (no carbon) acids.

The solvent can combine in long chains to form waxes and plastics.
Esters provide the pleasant fragrance and flavor of fruits and flowers.
Esters are calming, relaxing, and balancing essential oils.
Consequently, esters control the nervous system, making them antispasmodic.
Oil with high content of esters includes bergamot, valerian, and clary sage.

Aldehydes form from alcohols by removing hydrogen.
The solvent is highly reactive.
Aldehydes are an element of perfumes, dye, vitamins, hormones, and reducing sugars such as glucose.
Aldehydes have enjoyable fragrance.
Aldehydes can be vasodilators and are irritating to the skin.
Aldehydes exhibit anti-fungal, anti-inflammatory, disinfectant, sedative, and uplifting.
Consequently, aldehydes relieve stress while promoting relaxation.
Oils with high content are cinnamon, lemongrass, and cintronella.

Ketones are the result of oxidizing alcohols.
The solvent is very reactive.
Ketones exist in many sugars and are components of steroid hormones.
Ketones have a very distinctive fragrance.
Ketones exhibit mucus easing, cell/tissue regeneration, wound healing, and reducing scar properties.
They are sedative and calming.
Consequently, ketones promote new tissue growth and liquefy mucous.
Ketones exhibit anti-inflammatory response.
Prudence dictates caution during pregnancy .
Oils with high content are rosemary, red cedar, and wormwood.

Oxides such 1,8-cineol called eucalyptol are a usually a low percentage ingredient.
Oils with high content are eucalyptus globulus & radiata, helichrysum gymnocephalum, and niaouli.

Acids contain hydrogen attached to a simple molecule.
Acids are easily reactive to form salts.

Enough of that!
Suffice it to say, these chemicals give essential oils very valuable properties.
A brief understanding of the chemical recipe validates the use of essential oil for health and welfare.

GET A CHARGE OUT OF THAT

Not only do essential oils have chemical properties, they have electric-magnetic and frequency properties.

Well known physics affirms that every molecule, so every element, every mechanism, every biologic, every physical phenomenon which exists in the universe has a particular frequency (f) and electric-magnetic signature as observed in the unified energy equation.

The electrical charge of the diffused ions of oils may be negative or positive.
Negative ions interact with the parasympathetic nerve system.

The activity regulates sleep, rest, relaxation, and digestion.
Positive ions interact with the sympathetic nerve system.
The activity is energizing, strengthening, and recovering.

Nature promotes negative ion environment while electronic equipment promotes positive ion.
Negative ion oils include cedarwood, citrus, lavender, patchouli, and sandalwood.
Positive ions include clove, cypress, eucalyptus, frankincense, helichrysum, pine, rosemary, and ylang.

As far back as the 1920's, Dr. Royal Rife demonstrated the effect of frequency on organisms.
Unfortunately, with the advent of synthetic drugs after WWII, the research created less interest.
Because of their complexity, biologic organisms have both low frequency and high frequency responses.
Much of Dr. Rife's work involved the low frequency response of organisms.
Much of the research with oils is associated with high frequencies, measured in megahertz (MHz).

Professor Bruce Tainio was head of the Department of Agriculture at Eastern Washington University.
He developed a technique to monitor high frequency on some biological systems and essential oils.
In his high spectrum, higher frequency is better than a lower frequency as observed in the table.
The table is a compilation for some of his data. The values are in millions of cycles (MHz).

Brain	72-90
Healthy human body	62-68
Illness	<58
Cancer	<42
Death starts	< 25
Processed food	0 hz

Tainio observed essential oils have a high frequency range of 52 – 320 megahertz (MHz).
The lower range affects bones and structure, while the upper range affects the mental and spiritual.
Rose oil has the highest known frequency near 320 MHz.

Smelling coffee lowers the body frequency by 10 MHz, while sipping lowers the system by 15 MHz.
Negative thoughts lower the biologic frequency by 12 MHz, while positive rises by 10 MHz.
Prayer and meditation raise the response by 15 MHz.

As a point of reference, normal broadcast FM radio operates in the range of 88 – 108 MHz.
Old style television channel 2 occupied a nominal 54 MHz.

Products, including food and environmental, consists of chemicals, which are made of molecules.
Products which come in contact with the body are synthesized into energy including fuel.
The frequency of most products is lower than the nominal body frequency.
Not only do products have a frequency, but they also have a spin or polarity.
Some products positively increase the physical frequency while others decrease.

The equation for electric-magnetic and frequency energy are illustrated in the physics section.

VIBRATION COMMENTARY

A person with a new idea is a crank until the idea succeeds. — Mark Twain

At the risk of getting too technical, the following observations are important to the topic.
The discussion of frequency elicits an interesting set of responses from both religion and science.

Some religious use the ancient argument, if it is not physical, it is not real but otherworldly.
This understanding of physical is simply what they can observe.
Therefore, they often opine that people should not dabble is perceived occult, new-age vibration theory.
Granted some of the things stated on the internet are spooky.
Nevertheless, there is very good science backing up frequency responses.

Then the scientist who understands his area, but is limited in another area argues 'you can't do that.'
Consequently, frequency associated with oils or biology is summarily dismissed.
These well-educated souls again miss the nuances because the phenomenon is outside his area.

First, a clarification of terms is in order.
Vibrations are oscillations back and forth with a particular rhythm.
The rhythm is measured in changes or cycles in a second.
A cycle per second is called a Hertz (Hz), named for an early electrical researcher.

Well-known science affirms that all molecules vibrate at a frequency.
Scientists have observed the senses are associated with frequency and mass or electromagnetics.
Hearing is mass stimulated frequency nominally in the 20 – 20,000 Hz range.
Sight is electromagnetic frequency in the visible light spectrum of 400 – 790 THz (terahertz, 10^{12} Hz).
Smell has been associated with mass shape and frequencies in the infrared range.

Cold lasers in the same infrared frequency range are used for numerous healing methodologies.
Electrical signals are used to aid bone healing.
Radio frequencies have been used to kill agriculture pests.
Vibration (frequency) alters the chemical composition of wine.

Dr. Rife with Dr Johnson from USC medical school demonstrated frequency signals could kill cancer.
The research was widely publicized by leading regional newspapers and physicians in the 1930's.
Unfortunately, the equipment of the day was analog without the feedback of current technology.
So his frequency observations were sometimes later corrected.
Like so many pioneer researchers, his information was lost or destroyed.
Unfortunately, many modern efforts to replicate his work have been misdirected.

Our laboratory has long conducted research in high energy and natural energy phenomenon, including lightning and partial discharge.
Fifteen years ago, partial discharge looked like noise, but now is mainstream technology.
Lightning is still often regarded as an 'act of God', which cannot be controlled.
Our published research and application accepts the source as an 'act of God', but control is well established.

As an anecdotal example, during thunderstorms, I have watched lighting strike a radio tower three miles outside my office window.
I have observed as many as six strikes in one storm. Very cool.
Interestingly, the tower never quit operations.

Clearly, lightning can be controlled.
Numerous similar observations exist for structures including strikes to the Empire State building.

Because of our research, the lab is located in a remote farming area on the highest hill in the area.
No high-voltage transmission power lines are within miles.
The entire structure is a Faraday cage with an intricate grounding system.

Using broad-spectrum software defined radio, much of the electromagnetic frequencies can be analyzed.
As an initial check, rose essential oil was brought near the sensing antenna.
Although the process was tedious, high frequency disturbances were detected.
The spectrum display showed multiple peaks between 265.210 and 266.370 MHz.
The peaks disappeared with the removal of the oil from the near field.
For validity, the process was repeated numerous times on multiple occasions.

Although these were different from Prof. Tainio's frequency, the peaks are in the same range.
Because of the number of molecules in the oil, I would expect there to be even more frequencies.

A background noise level exists with any audio or electromagnetic frequency.
The oil emission was barely discernible above the background noise and at times was not detectable.
This is exactly the state of partial discharge analysis a few short years ago.
Even the software defined radio (SDR) used in the analysis was not available four years ago.
As sensors and analysis techniques improve, much more data will become accessible.

One additional comment is in order.
The background noise is simply the electromagnetic frequency emissions of activity in the universe.
Noise is information, which we have not yet identified or decoded.

Enough of that!
Suffice it to say electromagnetic and mass frequency responses impart to essential oils very valuable properties.
A brief understanding of the science validates the use of essential oil for health and welfare.

BACK TO THE BIBLE

We have veered into very technical, but still comprehendible areas to explain how oils work.
Now, look at the most ancient record to see oils and understand why they were used the way they were.

The Bible illustrates oils were used for cleaning, health, and aromatherapy (perfume).
Very specific blends invoked several different purposes.

Recall that the priests were knowledgeable about law, science, astronomy, medicine, and health.
The renaissance-man practice remained common through Rene Descartes in 1650, Isaac Newton in 1727, up to Marquis de Laplace in 1827.
These esteemed gentlemen were unabashed believers in the Creator and design of the creation.
Since Laplace, scientists have increasingly become specialists in increasingly small fields.
The specialization has limited their perception of the integrity of the universe.

Similarly, philosophers have moved from rational practicality to emotional haranguing in ivory towers. Very few of us polymath generalists continue to practice, research, and publish.

Tabernacle Cleaning Compound

Priests used a specific formulation of oils for tabernacle cleaning, not for putting on people.

> *Then the Lord said to Moses, "Take the following fine spices: 500 shekels of liquid myrrh, half as much (that is, 250 shekels) of fragrant cinnamon, 250 shekels of fragrant calamus, 500 shekels of cassia—all according to the sanctuary shekel—and a hin (about 250 shekels) of olive oil.*
> --Exodus 30:23-24 NIV

The spices were derived from resins and dried bark.
Two hundred fifty shekels was about 3.09 liters.
The conversion from weight to volume assumes a specific gravity of 0.97 for the oil.
The shekel of the sanctuary simply means the official weight, like stamps on gasoline pumps.

The ratio was 2 parts myrrh and cassia with 1 part cinnamon and calamus in 1 part olive oil.
This is clearly a precise recipe.

> *Make these into a sacred anointing oil, a fragrant blend, the work of a perfumer. It will be the sacred anointing oil. Then use it to anoint the tent of meeting, the ark of the covenant law, the table and all its articles, the lampstand and its accessories, the altar of incense, the altar of burnt offering and all its utensils, and the basin with its stand. You shall consecrate them so they will be most holy, and whatever touches them will be holy. "Anoint Aaron and his sons and consecrate them so they may serve me as priests.*
> --Exodus 30:25-30 NIV

Holy simply means exceptional, special, or separate.
The blend is a very effective disinfectant for cleansing the butcher and raw meat area.
Hence, the mixture was effective on surfaces and the priests clothing to maintain sanitary conditions.

> *Say to the Israelites, 'This is to be my sacred anointing oil for the generations to come. Do not pour it on anyone else's body and do not make any other oil using the same formula. It is sacred, and you are to consider it sacred. Whoever makes perfume like it and puts it on anyone other than a priest must be cut off from their people.' "*
> — Exodus 30:31-33 NIV

The ingredients are 'hot' oils, which mean they are strong irritants that burn the skin.
One drop of pure cinnamon has sent me scurrying to find a carrier to dilute the strong irritant.
The mixture was not suitable for human contact.
If an untrained person had the blend, he could potentially injure someone.

Diffuse Incense Compound

> *Then the Lord said to Moses, 'Take fragrant spices — gum resin (stacte, myrrh), onycha and galbanum — and pure frankincense, all in equal amounts, and make a fragrant blend of incense, the work of a perfumer. It is to be salted (tempered) and pure and sacred. Grind some of it*

to powder and place it in front of the ark of the covenant law in the tent of meeting, where I will meet with you. It shall be most holy to you.
— Exodus 30:34-36 NIV

The aromatic blend was potent incense.
Heating the resins drives the essential oils into the air.
The purpose was identical to contemporary diffusing of essential oils.
The aromatics were equivalent to spraying a room with original Lysol® to disinfect the hidden spaces.

The aromatics are effective disinfectants.
Onycha, also called benzoin, was a disinfectant in hospitals until WWII, replaced by patented synthetics.

Do not make any incense with this formula for yourselves; consider it holy to the Lord. Whoever makes incense like it to enjoy its fragrance must be cut off from their people.
— Exodus 30:37-38 NIV

Myrrh increases spiritual awareness and impacts hormones.
Onycha creates euphoria.
Galbanum aids in meditation and spiritual awareness.
Interestingly, the oil's frequency increases dramatically when mixed with frankincense and sandalwood.
Frankincense reduces brain noise, increases meditation and spiritual awareness, and enhances dreams.

All the essences create a 'high', so too much could be narcotic.
A little is great, too much is not.
Consequently, the blend was a controlled substance.

Personal Cleansing Compound
Leviticus 14 recites the procedure for cleansing skin conditions, leprosy, mold, and mildew.
Equal parts of cedarwood and hyssop were blended.
Cedarwood is one of the oils highest in sesquiterpenes, which assures oxygen to the pineal and pituitary.
Cedarwood is anti-fungal, anti-infectious, and antiseptic.
Hyssop consists of ketones, terpenes, phenols, and esters, which makes it a strong solvent.
Hyssop is anti-asthmatic, anti-cararrhal, anti-infectious, anti-inflammatory, anti-oxidant, anti-parasitic, antiseptic, and anti-viral.

The process was to anoint right ear, right thumb, and right toe; then pour the remainder over the head.
The locations are reflex points for parent emotions, fear of unknown block to learning, and addictions or bad habits respectively.
The individual was isolated for 7 days.
Then he shaved all hair from his body to clean any remaining contaminants.
The combination of disinfectant, isolation, and shaving is still an effective way to kill microbes.

Burnt offerings were simply barbecuing cloven-footed, cud-chewing meat for food.
Ascertaining the purpose of the other elements of the cleansing practice is not clear.
Obviously, the priests had an understanding of the use of oils and sanitary practices.

ESSENTIAL OIL CATEGORIES

Categorization of essential oils takes many forms.
Perhaps the most common involves the source, which includes flowers, herbs, and trees.
Further segmentation consists of the part producing the oil.

> Floral
> > Flowers
> Herbal
> > Leaves - spice
> > Seeds, berries
> > Roots
>
> Woody
> > Fruit rind - citrus
> > Resins, gum, sap, balsam
> > Wood bark

Nuts are fatty and not particularly aromatic.
Therefore, nuts seldom produce essential oils.

ESSENTIAL OIL PROPERTIES

The plants and essential oils noted in the Bible are in an earlier section.
A detail of each oil and plant part follows.
The chemicals, characteristics, and reported uses tell the importance of each essential oil.

Notice each essential oil reportedly has numerous effects.
Before considering any essential oils, be aware of its indications and contra-indications.

The chemistry percentages are typical and vary with growing and processing conditions.
The information derives from multiple sources.

The following information is simply an overview, is not comprehensive, or all-inclusive.
A thorough understanding of possible uses will reduce the risk of problems.
The information is research for educational purposes.
The information is not provided to diagnose, prescribe, or treat any disease or illness.

Understanding all the terms and details is not necessary to grasp the utility of the oil.

| Acacia / shittah / gum arabic / mimosa | Chemicals | anisaldehyde, benzoic acid, benzyl alcohol, butyric acid, coumarin, cresol, cuminaldehyde, decanal, eicosane, eugenol, farnesol, geraniol, 2-hydroxyacetophenone, methyleugenol, |

		methyl salicylate, nerolidol, palmitic acid, salicylic acid, and alpha-terpineol
acacia farnesiana	Character	demulcent, anti-inflammatory
flower, resin	Common uses	uplifting, calming, relieve stress
diffuse, topical	Possible other	fixative, anionic

Aloes/ sandalwood	Chemicals	sesquiterpene alcohol (<80%), sesquiterpene (<11%), sesquiterpene aldehyde (<3%), carboxylic acids
santalum album	Character	anti-depressant, anti-septic, anti-tumor, aphrodisiac, astringent, crosses blood brain barrier with oxygen, calming, sedative, tonic
heartwood & roots	Common uses	lumbago & sciatica, confusion, hemorrhoids, hiccups, laryngitis, multiple sclerosis, UV radiation, wrinkles
food additive, diffuse, neat	Possible other	cardiovascular, coughs, emotional balance, hormones, remove negative programming of cells, skin repair

Anise	Chemicals	phenolic ethers <95%, alcohols, phenols, aldehydes
pimpenella anisum	Character	anti-fungal, anti-septic, anti-spasmodic, analgesic, expectorant, estrogen-like, diuretic, heart stimulant, tonic, vermifuge
seed	Common uses	alkalosis, bronchitis, colitis, increase estrogen, PMS, flatulence
gras, diffuse, topical	Possible other	skin irritant, addictive narcotic

Balm / balsam / opopanax / sweet myrrh	Chemicals	sesquiterpenes, et al
Commiphora erythraea / opobalsamum	Character	anti-infectious, anti-inflammatory, anti-oxidant, anti-septic, anti-tumor, analgesic, astringent, tonic
resin	Common uses	cancer(particularly breast & prostate), diabetes, dysentery, fumigant, fungal

		issues (Candida, ringworm, eczema), Hasimoto's, hyperthyroidism, hepatitis, tooth/gum issues or infections, skin issues (chapped, cracked, impetigo, wrinkles, stretch marks), ulcer
food additive, diffuse, topical	Possible other	Caution photoxic

Bay	Chemicals	pinene, myrcene, limonene, linalool, chavicol, neral, terpineol, geranyl acetate, and eugenol
laurilus nobilis	Character	anti-oxidant, anti-septic
leaves	Common uses	reduce hair-loss, help confidence & courage & creativity, respiratory, stomach
food additive, diffuse, topical	Possible other	prophecy & divination, uplifting peace of mind

Calamus / cane	Chemicals	sesquiterpene ketones, aldehydes, phenol ether
acorus calamus	Character	antibiotic, antispasmodic, circulatory, cephalic, stimulant, nervine
roots	Common uses	nervous system stimulant, headaches, neuralgia, panic attacks, improving memory, reducing joint swelling, pain reliever
diffuse very dilute topical	Possible other	nervous complaints, vertigo, headaches, neuralgia, shock, epilepsy, panic attacks, dysentery

Cassia / Chinese cinnamon	Chemicals	cinnamic aldehyde(<85%), benzaldehyde, phenols(>7%): eugenol, chavicol; esters
cinnamomum cassia	Character	carminative, anti-diarrhea, anti-microbial, anti-emetic
bark, twigs, stalk	Common uses	colds, colic, dyspepsia, nausea, rheumatism, kidney, reproductive complaints
spice extreme irritant	Possible other	Caution with aromatherapy and topical since it is extreme irritant.

Cedarwood	Chemicals	sesquiterpenes(<90%): himachalenes(>55%),sesquiterpene alcohol(<40%), sesquiterpene ketones(20%)
cedrus atlantica	Character	anti-fungal, anti-infectious, anti-septic, anti-spasmodic, astringent, diuretic, emmenagogue, insect repellent, sedative, crosses blood brain barrier with oxygen
bark	Common uses	calming, cellulite, hair loss, tension, tuberculosis, urinary infection, ancient Egyptian mummification
diffuse dilute topical	Possible other	acne, anxiety, arthritis, congestion, cough, cystitis, dandruff, psoriasis, purification, sinusitis, skin diseases, water retention

Cinnamon	Chemicals	cinnamic aldehyde(<50%), benzaldehyde, phenols(<30%): eugenol, alcohols, sesquiterpenes
cinnamomum verum cinnamomum zeylan	Character	analgesic, anti-microbial, antispasmodic (anti-cholinergic), anti-inflammatory, anti-oxidant, aphrodisiac, astringent, cardiac, carminative, emmenagogue, insecticide, stimulant, stomachic, tonic, vermifuge
bark	Common uses	diabetes, diverticulitis, digestion, pneumonia, staph/MRSA, vaginal infection, warming, whooping cough
spice extreme irritant	Possible other	Yet to find a virus, bacteria, or fungus to survive it. infections, exhaustion, rheumatism, warts

Cistus / labdanum / rose of Sharon	Chemicals	monoterpenes(<65%>, alcohols, esters, ketones, aldehydes, acid
cistus ladanifer	Character	anti-bacterial, anti-hemorrhagic, anti-inflammatory, anti-microbial, anti-septic, anti-viral, astringent, diuretic, expectorant, tonic, immune stimulant, sympathetic nerves

gum	Common uses	sciatica, stop bleeding
food additive, diffuse, dilute topical	Possible other	boils, bronchitis, colds, rhinitis, urinary infections, stop bleeding in open wounds, wrinkles. anti: *Staphylococus aureus*, *Escherichia coli* and *Candida albicans*

Coriander	Chemicals	alcohols <80%, monoterpenes ,24%, esters, ketones, aldehydes
coriandrum sativum	Character	anti-bacterial, anti-fungal, anti-heumatic, anti-inflammatory, antimicrobial, anti-oxidant, anti-spasmodic
seed, leaves are cilantro	Common uses	aphrodisiac, blood sugar, lowers glucose, joint pain - arthritis, gout, fatigue, nervousness, constipation & digestion issues, hemorrhoids, neuralgia, measles
food additive, diffuse, topical	Possible other	stupefying in large dose, flavor wine & liqueurs

Cumin	Chemicals	monoterpenes <75%, aldehydes <60%, phenols, sesquiterpenes
cuminum cyminum	Character	anti-inflammatory, anti-tumoral, antioxidant, antiviral, a digestive aid, supports the liver and stimulates the immune system, stimulate appetite
seeds	Common uses	AIDS/HIV, cancer, diabetes, infectious disease, digestive issues
gras, diffuse, topical	Possible other	lymphatic congestion, morphine withdrawal

Cypress	Chemicals	monoterpenes <77%, sesquiterpene alcohols <15%, alcohols <9%, esters 5%
cupressus sempervirens	Character	anti-bacterial, anti-infectious, anti-microbial, anti-septic, hepatic, mucolytic, styptic, deodorant, diuretic, lymphatic & prostate decongestant, refreshing, sedative, vasoconstrictor
branches	Common	aneurysm, bunion, bursitis, carpal

| | uses | tunnel, cataracts, concussion, hemorrhoids, herniated disc, jock itch, Lou Gehrig's, muscle fatigue, nose bleed, Raunaud's, shingles, stroke, toxemia, tuberculosis, varicose veins |
| diffuse dilute topical | Possible other | asthma, strengthen capillary walls, reduce cellulite, circulatory, colds, strengthen connective tissue, spasmodic coughs, diarrhea, edema, energy, fever, gallbladder, bleeding gums, hemorrhaging, influenza, laryngitis, liver disorder, lung circulation, muscle cramps, nervous tension, ovarian cysts, increase perspiration, skin care, scar tissue, whooping cough, wounds. |

Dill	Chemicals	monoterpenes <65%, ketones <45%, ethers <11%
anethum graveolens	Character	anti-bacterial, anti-diabetic, anti-spasmodic, expectorant, lower glucose, pancreatic stimulant, promotes lactation
seed, whole plant	Common uses	cholesterol, indigestion, liver, painful periods
gras, diffuse, topical	Possible other	constipation, dyspepsia, flatulence, headaches, caution if susceptible to epilepsy

Fir – white / silver	Chemicals	monoterpenes <95%, esters <10%
abies alba	Character	anti-arthritic, anti-catarrhal, anti-oxidant, anti-septic, anti-tumoral, analgesic, expectorant, stimulant
needles	Common uses	anti-oxidant, cleaning bath/kitchen, furniture polish, muscle aches & fatigue
food additive, diffuse, topical	Possible other	deodorant, Christmas tree

| **Frankincense / olibanum** | Chemicals | monoterpenes <90%, sesquiterpenes <10%, alcohols <5% |
| *boswellia carteri* | Character | anti-catarrhal, anti-cancer, anti-depressant, anti-infectious, anti- |

		inflammatory, anti-septic, anti-tumoral, astringent, carminative, digestive, diuretic, emmenagogue, expectorant, immune stimulant, sedative, skin mature, tonic, uterine, vulnerary, wound healing, crosses blood brain barrier with oxygen
resin	Common uses	arthritis, asthma, brain injury, coma, concussion, confusion, coughs, depression, skin infection, inflammation, laryngitis, Lou Gehrig's, mental fatigue, moles, multiple sclerosis, Parkinson's, scarring, ulcer, warts, wrinkles
food additive, diffuse, dilute topical	Possible other	aging, allergies, bites (insect & snake), bronchitis, carbuncles, colds, diphtheria, gonorrhea, headaches, hemorrhaging, herpes, high blood pressure, jaundice, laryngitis, meningitis, nervous, prostate problems, pneumonia, respiratory, scarring, sciatica, sores, spiritual, staph, strep, stress, syphilis, tuberculosis, tension, tonsillitis, typhoid, wounds, warts.

Galbanum	Chemicals	monoterpenes <95% , sesquiterpene alcohols, esters, coumarins
ferula gummosa	Character	analgesic, anti-infectious, anti-inflammatory, anti-microbial, anti—septic, anti-spasmodic, anti-viral, diuretic, expectorant, insect bites/stings, pain-reliever, restorative, aging skin, tonic
resin from branches	Common uses	wounds, paralysis, muscle wasting(polyneuritis)
food additive, diffuse, dilute topical	Possible other	historical embalming

Henna / mehndi / camphire	Chemicals	1,4-naphthoquinone, tannins, gallic acid, flavonoids, lipids, sugars, triacontyl tridecanoate, mannitol, xanthones, coumarins (5alkyloxy 7-

		hydroxycoumarin), 2-3% resins, 5-10% tannic ingredients and up to 2% Lawsone (2hydroxy-1,4-naphthoquinone
lawsonia inermis	Character	anti-bacterial, anti-tumor, emmenagogue, rejuvenating, relaxant, stimulate hair growth
flowers	Common uses	dye tints skin, skin issues –leprosy & boils, induce menstruation & uterine contractions, meditation, cool body
topical and bath	Possible other	Avoid during pregnancy, no indication of skin irritation

Hyssop	Chemicals	ketones>58%, monoterpenes>25%, sesquiterpene <7%, phenols 4%, alcohols, esters, oxides
hyssopus officinalis	Character	anti-asthmatic, anti-catarrhal, anti-infectious, anti-inflammatory, anti-oxidant, anti-parasitic, anti-septic, anti-spasmodic, anti-viral, astringent, decongestant, diuretic, mucolytic, sedative
stems & leaves	Common uses	kidney stones, allergies, bruises, circulatory disorders, congestion, lack of energy, parasites, respiratory infections, viral infections
gras, diffuse, dilute topical	Possible other	Avoid with high blood pressure, pregnancy, & epilepsy

Juniper / gin	Chemicals	monoterpenes 50%, esters < 20%, ketones 19%, sesquiterpene <3%
juniperus osteosperma / communis	Character	anti-spasmodic, astringent, cleanser, detoxifier, diuretic, stimulant, tonic
berry	Common uses	skin diseases – acne & dermatitis, alcoholism, kidney stones, tinnitus, against contagious disease
gin ingredient, diffuse, topical	Possible other	coughs, depression, liver, aching muscles, stimulate uterine muscles, spiritual awareness

Mint / horsemint	Chemicals	ketones <70%, monoterpenes <30%, alcohols <10%, sesquiterpenes <5%, esters, oxides
Menthe longafolia	Character	diaphoretic, diuretic, stimulant, carminative, anti-spasmodic, nervine, sedative, nephritic, anti-emetic
herb	Common uses	soothing to nerves, stomach, kidneys, and bladder, vomiting and nausea of pregnancy, hemorrhoids
food additive, diffuse, topical	Possible other	condiment, milder than peppermint, preferable for infants

Myrrh / stacte	Chemicals	sesquiterpene <75%, furanoids <27%, ketones <20%, monoterpenes, aldehydes, acids, phenols
commiphora myrrha	Character	anti-infectious, anti-inflammatory, anti-oxidant, anti-septic, anti-tumor, analgesic, astringent, tonic
resin	Common uses	cancer (particularly breast & prostate), diabetes, dysentery, fungal issues (candida, ringworm, eczema), Hasimoto's, hyperthyroidism, hepatitis, tooth/gum issues or infections, skin issues (chapped, cracked, impetigo, wrinkles, stretch marks), ulcer
food additive, diffuse, dilute topical	Possible other	appetite, asthma, athlete's foot, candida, catarrh, coughs, eczema, digestion, dyspepsia, flatulence, fungal, gingivitis, hemorrhoids, prostate, ringworm, sore throats, wounds. Caution with pregnancy.

Myrtle	Chemicals	oxides 1,8 cineole <45%, monoterpenes <45%, esters <22%, alcohols <18%, aldehydes, phenols, furanoids
myrtus communis	Character	anti-bacterial, anti-inflammatory, anti-parasitic, anti-septic, anti-spasmodic, astringent, deodorizer; sinus & lung decongestant, expectorant & mucolytic; liver, prostate & thyroid stimulant
leaves	Common uses	skin irritations: acne, blemishes, bruises, oily, wrinkles, psoriasis, hemorrhoids; antiseptic for urinary tract

food additive, diffuse, dilute topical	Possible other	normalizing hormonal thyroid and ovaries, balancing hypothyroid; soothing respiratory

Narcissus / rose of Isaiah	Chemicals	benzyl acetate 24%, benzyl alcohol 21%, methyl benzoate, p-cresol, phenethyl alcohol, indole
narcissus tazetta	Character	anti-depressant, anti-septic, anti-spasmodic, aphrodisiac, expectorant, scar healing, astringent, sedative
flower	Common uses	asthma, cramps, convulsions, depression, fatigue, stimulate menstruation, skin
diffuse, topical	Possible other	

Onycha / benzoin	Chemicals	esters <70%, acids <30%-benzoic, cinnamic, aldehydes- vanillin, alcohols
styrax benzoin	Character	anti-inflammatory, antioxidant, anti-septic, astringent, deodorant, diuretic, expectorant, euphoric, sedative
resin	Common uses	open wounds, fixative; skin: cracked, acne, eczema, psoriasis; stimulating: mucus, circulation, expels gas, increases urine; respiratory
food additive, diffuse, dilute topical	Possible other	potent antiseptic & disinfectant. In alcohol, tincture of benzoin was predominant hospital antiseptic prior to patented, synthetic antiseptics.

Pine	Chemicals	monoterpenes <80%, sesquiterpenes <12%, alcohols, esters, aldehydes, phenols
pinus sylvestris	Character	anti-bacterial, anti-microbial, anti-neuralgic, anti-septic, anti-viral, expectorant, stimulant to adrenal, circulatory, nervous
	Common uses	gout, sinusitis, bronchial, colds, coughs, cuts, cystitis, fatigue, feet sweating, gout, lice, scabies, stress, urinary infection

food additive, diffuse, topical	Possible other	increases blood pressure, stimulate adrenals can circulatory, first aid

Rue	Chemicals	2-Undecanone or 'rue ketone' 47 %, and 2-nonanone 19 %
ruta graveolens	Character	stimulant, emmemagogue, anti-spasmodic, anti-septic, anthelmintic (germicide), nervine, carminative, disinfectant, anti-rheumatic, tonic, emetic, anti-venomous, rubifacient, counter-irritant, diuretic
Herb, leaves	Common uses	uterus & ovaries, stomach, colic, typhoid & malaria fever, vertigo, heart palpitations, sciatica, rheumatism, eye inflammation, epilepsy,
food additive, diffuse, topical	Possible other	most bitter herb, use very small dose, abortifacient

Saffron / kesar	Chemicals	safranal 70%, 2-hydroxy-4,4,6-trimethyl-2,5-cyclohexadien-1-one
crocus sativus	Character	anti-septic, anti-carcinogenic, anti-mutagenic, anti-inflammatory, antioxidant, immune system modulating
flower	Common uses	oily skin, acne, cuts, inhibit cancer cell
flavoring agent, diffuse, topical	Possible other	removing stress, annoyance, negative thoughts, depression, mental fatigue

Spikenard	Chemicals	sesquiterpenes <50%, monoterpenes <45%, alcohols, ketones <10%, phenolic aldehyde, coumarins; 1,8cineol; acids
nardostachys jatamansi	Character	anti-bacterial, anti-fungal, anti-inflammatory, deodorant, relaxant, immune stimulant
roots	Common uses	insomnia, menstrual issues such as PMS, heart arrhythmia, nervous tension, regenerating the skin
diffuse, dilute topical	Possible other	allergic skin reactions, flatulent indigestion, insomnia, migraine, nausea,

		rashes, stress, tachycardia, tension, slow healing wounds anti: candida, staph

Terebinth / pistachio	Chemicals	monoterpenes 55%
pistacia terebinthus	Character	anti-bacterial, anti-catarrhal, anti-septic, analgesic, insecticide, warming
leaves	Common uses	digestion, dissolve gall stones, genital tract, gout, muscular aches , neuralgia, rheumatic pain, sciatica
food additive, diffuse, topical	Possible other	food processing, preservation

Wormwood / absinthe /bitters	Chemicals	thujone, monoterpene alcohols, sesquiterpene lactone
artemesia judiaca	Character	tonic, anthelmintic, vermifuge, stomach, stimulant, febrifuge, hepatic, anti-septic, nervine, anti-venomous, anti-bilious, carminative
herb	Common uses	roundworms, dyspepsia, diarrhea, bile and liver troubles, epilepsy, debility, melancholia, jaundice, nausea, morning sickness, intermittent fevers, gout, rheumatism, swelling, sprains
food additive, diffuse, topical	Possible other	second most bitter herb, used with alcoholic beverage

Numerous sources provided information and not all agree.
If you find any error or mistake, please notify the publisher.

The gums and resins are very thick.
 Diffusing may need dilution with lemon or other oils.

Interestingly, this group of oils represents properties and uses for most all common oils.
The exception is citrus oils, which did not exist in the Middle East at the time of scribing the Bible.
Citrus was a Chinese fruit, so it was not available in the Levant.

INTERESTING BLENDS

Two blends of oils have colorful stories.
The names used are the most commonly recognized and are the property of Young Living®.

Other companies offer similar blends with their own names.

The compelling story is a group of spice traders from India were in Europe during the Black Plague.
The people were afraid to touch the bodies of victims.
Aware of the properties of vinegar and spices, the merchants rubbed their body with the aromatics.
With their protection, the thieves proceeded to loot the homes and bodies of plague victims.
When caught, the king released the thieves in exchange for their secret of protection.

Thieves® is only one of the numerous formulations reportedly used by the spice traders.
The ingredients are consistent across the blends; however, the quantities vary.
My version of the blend is 2 clove, 1 cinnamon, 1 lemon, 1 eucalyptus, 1 rosemary.
Dilute with 1 drop of the blend to 4 drops of carrier.
The formula is highly effective as a cleaning, disinfecting product and anti-microbial.

Rosemary can elevate blood pressure, so its use should be cautionary for those with hypertension.

Valor® is one of the formulations reportedly used by Roman soldiers to bolster courage.
Several variations of the formula are available.
One version contains 15 parts blue spruce, 7 parts frankincense, 6 parts blue tansy, 2 parts balsam fir or rosewood with 20% almond oil carrier.
The fusion is effective in relieving the back and spine, in my experience.

BLOOD PRESSURE

Those factors, which become issues, are the things in which we are most interested.
Blood pressure is a common consequence of many bodily challenges.
Allopathic medicines are experimentally tried until something sort of works on the symptoms.
When I was still an active pilot, in an annual physical my blood pressure was elevated.
The nurse wisely cautioned me about taking the myriad versions of medication.
Diet, nutrition, and awareness have controlled the issue within very acceptable limits for 25 years.

Published data lists the following oils apparent effect on blood pressure.
Raise (avoid if hypertensive): hyssop, rosemary, sage, thyme, and peppermint.
Lower (avoid if hypotensive):   ylang ylang, marjoram, eucalyptus, lavender.

HORMONES

Hormones are communications signals, which control body functions.
The chemicals in essential oils actively influence hormones.
The oils identified are not the only ones, which drive these critical systems.
In our culture, we seek treatments to make things to go up or to make go down.
Interestingly many oils are balancing, meaning the chemicals move the issue as needed.

Clary sage balances estrogen.
Clary also reduces cortisol by as much as 36% in some studies, and improves thyroid (TSH).
The oil has anti-depressant response on mood.

Thyme improves progesterone production for women and men.

Sandalwood has a fabulous scent and increases testosterone.
Sandalwood has a reputation for aphrodisiac and improving impotence. What is not to like?

Rose improves serotonin and other neuro-transmitters (-peptides), which are the feel good drivers.

Lavender and chamomile lower cortisol by reducing stress, which aids in disease recovery.

Frankincense improves thyroid and autoimmune response, while reducing inflammation.
Frankincense is perhaps the most utilitarian health assisting essential oil.
If I had only one essential oil in my kit, frankincense is it.

Rosemary reduces DHT, which reduces hair loss and reduces prostate issues for men.

Myrrh reportedly helps hypothyroid issues.
Myrrh enhances uterine contractions and lowers blood sugar.

MODERATION

Let your moderation be known unto all men. The Lord is at hand. – Philippians 4:5 NKJV

Too much or too little food or drink is unhealthy.
Overindulgence in virtually any activity is deleterious.
Since essential oils have a complex recipe of very powerful chemicals, moderation is extremely important.
In moderation, the oils are very pleasant and helpful.
In excess, the oils can be sensitizing or potentially noxious.

Alternate authorities may disagree with an over-abundance of caution.
Since this is an educational document, both the benefits and some cautions are noted.
Furthermore, knowing the published information is important when evaluating an oil for use.

Do not ingest any essential oil without adequate knowledge and training.

Variations in methodology cause oil from different sources to be very different or have toxic residue.
Use only purest, therapeutic grade, from reputable sources.
In my research and experience, competitive priced retail brands are not as effective.
There is a reason for the price.

Further, mixing of lesser quality oils can create strange results.
I have mixed less expensive lemon and eucalyptus in water and produced an insoluble white crystal salt.
Just saying!

The International Fragrance Association (IFRA) is a trade group, which uses essential oils, components, and other materials in the manufacture of perfume, cleansers, and other household products.

Because the products are used by the public with little training or skill, caution is in order.
Hence, the IFRA sets usage standards.
For the essential oils ingredients, which are more harmful if over indulged, IFRA has a banned list.
For the oils components, which are irritants or requires limits on quantity, IFRA has a restricted list.
The annexes contain both lists.

Many of these oils have been safely employed in various forms for eons.
Just be aware!

Since oils are very potent, the bottom of the feet is often the safest place for application on skin.
The area is less sensitive, but still allows absorption.

If used on the skin, with very few exceptions, dilution of all oils is advised.
Reference Guide for Essential Oils by Higley gives recommendations for dilution ratios.
The book also identifies oils suitable for internal use and generally regarded as safe (GRAS) by FDA.

I tend to dilute even more, since so many molecules are present in one drop of the oils.
Several other sources have variations on similar information.
A later table illustrates published and commonly accepted dilution quantities.

Tisserand wrote, "There is no documented evidence of inhaled allergy to any essential oil, the only existing evidence relates to [synthetic] fragrances."

WHY MODERATION

Irritants cause rash, itching, stinging, or tingling.
Sensitizers given enough exposure may become allergenic and cause cross-sensitization to other oils.

Some authors argue once an allergy sets in, then the allergy is for a lifetime.
While it may be true for allopathic medicine, that opinion does not stand the test of validated reality.
The opinion explicitly affirms healing cannot exist. Poppycock.

Allergic reaction depends on numerous things including general health, age, and environment.
Appropriate corrective action continues to mediate allergenic effects.
As a minimum, address the liver, adrenals, pituitary, and inflammation.

Preferred for use of the sensitizing oils is in diffusers, rather than topically.
Application to the skin should be limited and then only if the oil is effectively diluted.

Conifers (pinaceae) and expressed citrus oils become stronger with age greater than 6 months.
What is common between these oils?
Monoterpenes - see how the chemistry provides increases understanding?
Distilled versions are less allergenic than other preparations.

The very thing that makes the oil very effective is the same thing that may make the oil noxious.

Phenol is an excellent antiseptic, anti-bacterial, and disinfectant.

Phenols include eugenol, thymol, and carvacrol, among myriad others.
Phenols cause most skin sensitivity from essential oils.
Use in low concentration for a short time, since an overworked liver may allow potentially toxic buildup.
Dilute appropriately and avoid sensitive areas.

For example, clove oil is the greatest anti-oxidant known.
Anti-oxidants are consequently anti-inflammatory.
Eugenol, which is a phenol, is present in the oil, burns the skin if undiluted, and is potentially toxic in larger doses.
Are we going to cancel Christmas because of clove? Of course not.

In herbal form or as a food, toxicity is difficult since you will not eat enough to cause issues.
However, oils are extremely concentrated.

A little is good, a lot is not.

Heed the advice.
It took me four months to mitigate the hyper-sensitization of certain undiluted oils.
Am I an educated scientific user? Do I use therapeutically? Absolutely! IN MODERATION...

DILUTION CHART

The information relies on work by Dr. Kurt Schnaubelt, PhD and Robert Tisserant.
The general guidelines give basic information about percentage of oil to use for different circumstances.
By no means are these specific rules.

% EO	Circumstances
0.5	'hot' oils, like cinnamon
1	children, elderly, sensitive skin
2 - 3	daily skin care
10 - 25	short-term use
neat	localized like mosquito bites, burns, bruise

The next table shows the drops of essential oil needed to produce the percentage in carrier oil.
Drop size will vary with the oil viscosity and the size of dropper.
Use the standard conversion:
        30 drops = 1 ml = 0.203 tsp.

Carrier	Drops of essential oil					
	1%	2%	3%	5%	10%	25%
10 ml / 2 tsp	3	6	9	15	30	75

In a bath, disperse the drops of oil in an agent such as liquid castile soap or Epsom salt.
Oil without the dispersant obviously does not dilute easily in water, and will form globules.

If too much oil contacts the skin, causing irritation, place carrier oil on the inflamed area.
The carrier will dilute the essential oil.
Water does nothing but spread the oil, making matters worse.

Essential oil is a hydrocarbon chemical.
So, the oil will dissolve / degrade plastics and is flammable.

WHAT'S THE RISK?

The following tables illustrate potential negative effects from overuse of some components of oils.

Dr. Kurt Schnaubelt wrote, "To get out from underneath these layers of trumped-up concerns, the whole safety and toxicity discussion needs to be turned upside down. Instead of perpetrating mantras about imaginary dangers, the inherently benign nature of essential oils needs to be recognized."

The basis for toxicity in the table is often a single component.
The components are isolated, allowing the creation of a synthetic concoction from petroleum distillates.
However, the essential oil is a complex recipe where many chemicals interact.
Generally, complete oil is less of a problem than the isolated ingredients.

The oils are orders of magnitude safer than synthetic petroleum based substitutes.
Having worked in the petrochemical industry for a long lifetime, to my recollection all petroleum distillates are toxic.
The crude oil raw material is not an environmental toxin.
As a matter of principle, crude oil is a benign cleanser allowing no microbes to exist.
However, the fractionation of petroleum does create hazardous chemicals.
Similarly, essential oils are safe in moderation, although individual components can be harmful.

The only credible record I have found about the potential toxicity of essential oil is from 1993.
Hartnoll, et al, reported in the *Archives of Disease*.
A 2-year-old boy 'nearly died' after taking between 5 and 10 ml of oil of cloves.

Note several things about the report.
Clove oil is one of the hottest oils known with very high phenol content, which makes a great anti-oxidant.
The quantity was 2/3 of a standard dropper bottle.
The child was very young.
In spite of all these extremes, the effect was serious, but not fatal.
The report goes a long way to validate the safety of essential oils, even in extreme amounts.

As noted earlier, consider the statistics from American Association of Poison Control Centers.
Available published documents show NO serious or fatal poisonings as a result from essential oils.

NOW A LITTLE PHYSICS

A chiropractic doctor friend asked me to give the equations for why biofeedback works.

The same relationships apply to essential oils.
The section is oriented more to the physics than chemistry.
The section explains the earlier discussion of electric-magnetic and frequency response.

Although not reserved for scientists and mathematicians, the section veers in that direction.
Regardless, just looking through the discussion gives a grasp of the science.

The equations for the biofeedback system are from the unified field equation.
The fundamental measure for performance of any system is energy.
The complete relationship is a summation of the mass-diffusion, electric-magnetic, and frequency energy.

$$E = \frac{m\,D}{t_t} + \frac{\varphi\,q}{t_t} + h_p f$$

Where: E = energy, m = mass, D = diffusion, φ = magnetic flux, q = electric charge, f = frequency, h = Planck's constant, and t = cyclic time.
Frequency is waves (w) over cyclic time.
Diffusion defines the space-time continuum by the volume-gradient over a seasonal-time rate.
The three volume vectors include lever-arm ray rotation, wavelength motion, and displacement respectively.
At the light transition boundary, diffusion cyclic-time rate becomes the c^2 of Einstein's relationship.

$$D = \frac{b_{rs} \times d_t \cdot s_r}{t_r\,s_r}$$

Every element, every mechanism, every biologic, every physical phenomenon which exists in the universe has a particular frequency (f) and electric-magnetic signature as observed in this equation.

The energy operates as a feedback loop.
An outside stimulus provokes a system (1) feed-forward to cause a (2) response or effect.
The (3) feed-back compensates with an adjustment to the stimulus effect.

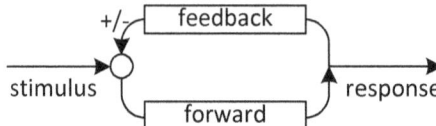

The general equation for the feedback loop is the classical relationship.

$$\frac{Response}{Simulus} = \frac{Forward}{1 + Forward * (\pm)\,Feedback}$$

In a bio-feedback system, the forward element is the energy defined in the first equation.
The feedback is the biological effect using the mental process.
Notice in the equation that feedback can be positive or negative. If the feedback is positive, then the response is stronger.
If the feedback is negative, then the response is weaker.

Well known science measures biological functions with electrical energy.

Brain waves use electro-encephalogram (EEG), muscle response uses electro-myogram (EMG), and heart function uses electro-cardiogram (EKG).
A cat scan is an image of electromagnetic waves from the brain or other organ.
An MRI is a magnetic resonance imaging of the electromagnetic frequency response.
The signals becomes stronger or weaker based on how the bio function is working.

Now consider the specific application of bio-feedback for 'muscle testing'.
Just as described, the mass energy becomes weaker if there is a negative feedback, and becomes stronger with positive feedback.

Similarly, 'witching', 'divining rods', or 'dowsing' operates with the same equations.
As written by Dr. S.W. Tromp in 1949, in this case, the mind thinks on the target.
When the biological filter of the mind matches (resonates with) the electric-magnetic and frequency energy of the target, then the mass of the rods will move.

Earlier discussion involved the frequency and electrical-magnetic signature of oils.
This brief monograph shows the equations and the feedback process for that and other discussions.

There is no magic, no oouh-oouh spirits, and no wizardry to bio-feedback systems. It is just physics.

OIL SOURCES & SUPPLIERS

The essential oil sources listed are reputable companies with quality oils, which we have used.
Commonly available brands, which I have evaluated, do not appear to be up to these.

Young Living® is a MLM distributor. Dr. D. Gary Young, one of the founders, has perhaps done more to promote understanding of essential oils than any other contemporary person has.

dōTERRA® is the second major MLM distributor.

Native American / Rocky Mountain® is a credible on-line distributor, with a real person on the phone, if needed.

Hopewell Essential Oils®, formerly Heritage Oils, is a small, independent, family business.
Their website gives information about the date and chemical composition of each batch.
Customer support and pricing has been excellent.
The quality, color, and aromatic potency have been greater than other equivalent oils we have analyzed.
Other knowledgeable users interviewed have independently affirmed similar observations.

REFERENCE TABLES IN ANNEX

Several tables are included as Annexes to provide more detailed and specific information.

References denote recent documents identified as significant contributions to facts in the paper.
Representative References is a partial tabulation of the numerous mentions of essential oils in the Bible.
IFRA Banned identifies components of oils, when isolated can cause noxious effects.
IFRA Restricted classifies components, which can contribute to irritating effects.
Other Cautionary limns essential oils that potentially can create undesirable issues.
GRAS tabulates numerous plants generally regarded as safe for consumption.

Explanations of the data in the tables give limitations of its applicability.

LEGAL STUFF

As indicated in the front cover, the information is copyrighted to control its integrity.
However, you may freely use all or some of the information, if not modified.

All we know is built on what we have learned from others, then enhanced in our own way.
The phenomenon of oils is available, natural elements, not patented surrogates.
Likewise, making knowledge about the oils freely available is desirable.

A note about the professions is in order to clarify any potential misunderstandings.
Physicians are highly skilled individuals trained to diagnose and treat patients according to a protocol.
Scientists, including engineers, develop the technology behind medicine.
Individuals with advanced degrees typically do research before technology or protocols are developed.
All skills are needed. One is not better than the other. The skill sets are just different.

The information in this manuscript is research for educational purposes.
It is not provided to diagnose, prescribe, or treat any disease or illness.
The author accepts no responsibility for such use.

RESEARCH

There is no magic, no oouh-oouh spirits, and no wizardry to essential oils. It is just science.

Research by,

Dr. Marcus O. Durham, PhD, ThD
Sr. Principal Analyst

THEWAY Labs
Laboratories/Failure Analysis/Energy Consultants
Electrical, Petro-Chemical, Natural
www.ThewayLabs.com

Life Fellow, Institute of Electrical & Electronics Engineers
Life Fellow, American College of Forensic Examiners Int'l
Life Sr. Member, Society of Petroleum Engineers
Diplomate, Am Board of Forensic Engineering &Tech
Licensed Electrical Contractor
Licensed Commercial Radiotelephone & Amateur Extra
Licensed Commercial Instrument Pilot, member AOPA
Cert Fire & Explosion Inv. & Cert Vehicle Fire Inv., NAFI
Certified Homeland Security, ABCHS
Registered Investigator, ABRI
Conservationist & Natural Energy researcher
Life member Phi Kappa Phi; Tau Beta Pi, Eta Kappa Nu
Author–15 books & over 150 scientific articles/papers
Richard H. Kaufmann Medal – IAS / IEEE
Professor Emeritus, University of Tulsa
Former Dean, Southwest Biblical Seminary

REFERENCES

Multiple references provided information over the years.
The information is a compilation largely based on experience and research.
Other than myriad oil documents over the decades, the key recent documents are noted.

Dr. Josh Axe, DNM, DC, CNS. *King's Medicine Cabinet,* https://draxe.com/, retrieved 04/02/2016.

Dr. Josh Axe, DNM, DC, CNS. "Top 3 Essential Oils to Balance Hormones Naturally", https://draxe.com/essential-oils-for-hormones, retrieved 6/16/16.

Dr. John R. Christopher, ND, MH. *School of Natural Healing*, Christopher Publications, Box 412, Springville, UT, 2014.

Marcus O. Durham, PhD, ThD. *Unified Field in One Energy Equation,* Tulsa: Realm Research, 2011, ISBN 978-1467950701.

Marcus O. Durham, PhD, ThD, and Robert A. Durham, PhD. "Does a Unified Energy Equation Contain the Higgs Field?" *IEEE Access*, Volume 1, New York, August 2, 2013.

Essential Oils Desk Reference, Essential Science Publishing, compiler, Lehi, UT.

Bo Jensen, MSc, http://www.bojensen.net/EssentialOilsEng/EssentialOils.htm, retrieved 7/10/2016

Hartnoll, G; Moore, D; Douek, D (1993). "Near fatal ingestion of oil of cloves". Archives of Disease in Childhood 69 (3): 392–3. doi:10.1136/adc.69.3.392. PMC 1029532. PMID 8215554

Connie & Alan Higley. *Reference Guide for Essential Oils,* Abundant Health, Spanish Fork, UT, 14th edition.

Nan Martin, LSHC-CRTS. "The Chemistry of Essential Oil Reveals Aromatherapy as a True Science!" Experience-Essential-Oils.com LLC, retrieved 6/16/16.

Kurt Schnaubelt, PhD. *The Healing Intelligence of Essential Oils*, Healing Arts Press, 2011.

David M. Stewart, PhD, DNM. *The Chemistry of Essential Oils*, Care Publications, Marble, MO, 2013.

David Stewart, PhD. *Healing Oils of the Bible*, Care Publications, Marble, MO, 2015.

Robert Tisserand & Rodney Young, PhD. *Essential Oil Safety: A Guide for Health Care Professionals,* Elsevier Health Sciences UK, 2nd Edition 2014.

The following supplier websites provided valuable information.

http://hopewelloils.com
http://www.essentialoils.co.za
http://www.rockymountainoils.com

ANNEXES

REPRESENTATIVE REFERENCES

Representative oil references: the list is by no means complete or exhaustive.

CALAMUS Exodus 30:23	HYSSOP Exodus 12:22 Leviticus 14:4, 6, 49, 51,52
CEDAR-WOOD Leviticus 14:4, 6, 49, 51, 52	Numbers 19:6, 18 1Kings 4:33 Psalm 51:7
CINNAMON Exodus 30:23 Proverbs 7:17 Song of Solomon 4:14 Revelation 18:13	John 19:29 Hebrew 9:19 JUNIPER Job 30:4
CORIANDER Exodus 16:31 Numbers 11:17	MYRRH Genesis 37:25, 43:11 Exodus 30:23 Esther 2:12
FRANKINCENSE Exodus 30:34 Leviticus 2:1, 2, 15, 16, 5:11, 6:15, 24:7 Numbers 5:15 1Chronicles 9:29 Nehemiah 13:5 Song of Solomon 3:6, 4:6, 14 Matthew 2:11 Revelation 18:13	Psalm 45:8 Proverbs 7:17 Song of Solomon 1:13, 3:6, 4:6, 14, 5:1, 5, 13 Matthew 2:11 Mark 15:23 John 19:39 MYRTLE Nehemiah 8:15 Isaiah 41:19, 55:13
GALBANUM Exodus 30:34	SPIKENARD Song of Solomon 1:12, 4:13, 14 Mark 14:3

	John 12:3

IFRA BANNED

This is a precautionary list, which shows possible side effects of a component in certain oils under extreme conditions.
The oils are the IFRA banned list.
The list information derives from several sources.
MODERATION: Avoid prolonged use and high doses.

Name	Scientific	Irritant	Use	Potential Oil Effect
Cade /prickly juniper	juniperus oxycedrus	Thujone, pinene		carcinogenic
Calamus -F	acorus calamus	asorone	nerves, headache, vertigo	oral convulsions, carcinogenic
Costus root	saussurea costus	zingiber		sensitizer
Elecampane oil	inula helenium	camphor	Respiratory, lung	sensitizer
Fig leaf absolute	ficus carica			sensitizer
Horseradish	cochlearia armoracia	allyl isothiocyanate	spice, coughs	irritant
Mustard	brassica nigra	allyl isothiocyanate not in dry seeds	spice	
Peru balsam	myroxylon var. pereirae		can lead to systemic reactions to common spices	strong sensitizer (distilled allowed)
Sassafras -F	sassafras albidum	safrole	rheumatism, gout	carcinogenic <
Savin - E	juniperus sabina	sabinene, sabinol , sabinyl acetate		abortifacient, irritant
Oriental sweetgum	liquidambar orientali		Skin, flavor	sensitizer
Tea absolute	thea sinensis			sensitizer
Verbena oil	lippia citriodora / aloysia triphylla		flavor	sensitizer
Wormseed - E	chenopodium ambrosioides		expel round & hook worms	toxin liver, heart, kidney
Wormwood	artemisio absinthium	thujone, sabinyl acetate	absinthe / bitters in drink	abortifacient, hallucinations, neurotoxin

< indicates even small amounts can cause the problem.
E indicates EU banned, F indicates FDA banned.

As is readily observed, the list contains numerous products, which are routinely used.
I really enjoy mustard and ground horseradish.

The food is very stimulating and pungent, but the quantity of oil ingested is limited.

When I was young, my paternal grandmother would harvest wild sassafras root.
Sassafras tea was a popular drink. Dad would limit the amount. The key is a tea was highly diluted.
Before the negative publicity, sassafras was the flavoring ingredient of root beer, another favorite drink.

The effect of wormwood is the same as any abuse of alcohol.

IFRA RESTRICTED

This is a precautionary list, which shows possible irritating side effects of ingredients in certain oils.
The oils are the IFRA restricted list.
The list information derives from several sources.
MODERATION: Avoid prolonged use and high doses.

Name	Scientific	Irritant	Use	Potential Oil Effect
Angelica root oil	angelica archangelica			phototoxic
Bergamot oil	citrus bergamia		citrus	phototoxic
Bitter orange oil	citrus aurantium		citrus	phototoxic
Cassia	cinnamomum cassia	cinnamic aldehyde	spice, digestive	sensitizer
Cinnamon bark	cinnamomum zeylanicum	cinnamic aldehyde	spice	sensitizer
Cumin oil	cuminum cyminum			phototoxic
Grapefruit oil	citrus paradisi		citrus	phototoxic
Lemon oil	citrus limon		citrus	phototoxic
Lime oil	citrus aurantifolia		citrus	phototoxic
Tagetes oil/absolute	tagetes minuta			phototoxic
Oak moss absolute/resinoid	evernia prunastri			sensitizer
Pinaceae oils	pinaceae mugo, p. nigra, p. pinaster, p. sylvatica		pine	sensitizer
Rue oil	ruta graveolens			sensitizer
Verbena absolute	lippia citriodora / aloysia triphylla			sensitizer
Tree moss absolute	(pseudeo) evernia furfuracea			sensitizer

Avoid phototoxic on an area of skin, which will be exposed to sun within 12 hours.
As is readily observed, the list contains numerous products, which are routinely used.
Cassia is one of the common cinnamons, which is a routinely consumed spice.
The citrus oils are excellent cleansers, disinfectants, and room fresheners.
A little bergamot tea or lemon tea is pleasing to the palette.

OTHER CAUTIONARY

This is a precautionary list, which shows possible side effects of certain components in certain other oils.
Other than wintergreen (birch), these items are less commonly used.
Wintergreen is aspirin, when used appropriately is very beneficial.
Wintergreen is also a flavoring.
My maternal grandfather used clear camphor for anything that did not move.

Name	Scientific	Irritant	Use	Potential Oil Effect
Almond (bitter)	prunus amygdalus	cyanide	flavor	lethal <
Boldo	peumus boldus		herb	convulsions <
Camphor, brown or yellow - E	cinnamomum camphora	safrole	White is ok. infections, respiratory	oral toxic
Mugwort	artemisia vulgaris			abortifacient, neurotoxin
Pennyroyal	mentha pulegium	puegone	menstrual	abortifacient, liver & lung <
Rue	ruta graveolens	methyl nonyl ketone	herbal	abortifacient, neurotoxin, phototoxic
Tansy	tanacetum vulgare	thujone	perfumery	neurotoxic, irritant
Thuja	thuja occidentalis	thujone		abortifacient, poison, neurotoxin
Wintergreen	gaultheria procumbens	methyl salicylate	aspirin	irritant, toxin

< indicates even small amounts can cause the problem.

GRAS

The Food and Drug Administration has published a list of plants products which are generally regarded as safe (GRAS) for food use.
As noted earlier, food consumption keeps down the quantity of oil ingested.
A significant fact is this agency has approved certain plants for food, while other groups restrict usage.
Go figure.
Reiterating, oils are generally safe when used in moderation.
The absence of an oil from the list certainly does not imply the oil is unhealthy or should not be used.
The list is taken directly from Code of Federal Regulations Title 21, Chapter 1, Subchapter B.

Common name	Botanical name of plant source
Alfalfa	Medicago sativa L.
Allspice	Pimenta officinalis Lindl.
Almond, bitter (free from prussic acid)	Prunus amygdalus Batsch, Prunus armeniaca L., or Prunus persica (L.) Batsch.
Ambrette (seed)	Hibiscus moschatus Moench.
Angelica root	Angelica archangelica L.
Angelica seed	Do.
Angelica stem	Do.
Angostura (cusparia bark)	Galipea officinalis Hancock.

Anise	Pimpinella anisum L.
Asafetida	Ferula assa-foetida L. and related spp. of Ferula.
Balm (lemon balm)	Melissa officinalis L.
Balsam of Peru	Myroxylon pereirae Klotzsch.
Basil	Ocimum basilicum L.
Bay leaves	Laurus nobilis L.
Bay (myrcia oil)	Pimenta racemosa (Mill.) J. W. Moore.
Bergamot (bergamot orange)	Citrus aurantium L. subsp. bergamia Wright et Arn.
Bitter almond (free from prussic acid)	Prunus amygdalus Batsch, Prunus armeniaca L., or Prunus persica (L.) Batsch.
Bois de rose	Aniba rosaeodora Ducke.
Cacao	Theobroma cacao L.
Chamomile flowers, Hungarian	Matricaria chamomilla L.
Chamomile flowers, Roman or English	Anthemis nobilis L.
Cananga	Cananga odorata Hook. f. and Thoms.
Capsicum	Capsicum frutescens L. and Capsicum annuum L.
Caraway	Carum carvi L.
Cardamom seed (cardamon)	Elettaria cardamomum Maton.
Carob bean	Ceratonia siliqua L.
Carrot	Daucus carota L.
Cascarilla bark	Croton eluteria Benn.
Cassia bark, Chinese	Cinnamomum cassia Blume.
Cassia bark, Padang or Batavia	Cinnamomum burmanni Blume.
Cassia bark, Saigon	Cinnamomum loureirii Nees.
Celery seed	Apium graveolens L.
Cherry, wild, bark	Prunus serotina Ehrh.
Chervil	Anthriscus cerefolium (L.) Hoffm.
Chicory	Cichorium intybus L.
Cinnamon bark, Ceylon	Cinnamomum zeylanicum Nees.
Cinnamon bark, Chinese	Cinnamomum cassia Blume.
Cinnamon bark, Saigon	Cinnamomum loureirii Nees.
Cinnamon leaf, Ceylon	Cinnamomum zeylanicum Nees.
Cinnamon leaf, Chinese	Cinnamomum cassia Blume.
Cinnamon leaf, Saigon	Cinnamomum loureirii Nees.
Citronella	Cymbopogon nardus Rendle.
Citrus peels	Citrus spp.
Clary (clary sage)	Salvia sclarea L.
Clover	Trifolium spp.
Coca (decocainized)	Erythroxylum coca Lam. and other spp. of Erythroxylum.
Coffee	Coffea spp.
Cola nut	Cola acuminata Schott and Endl., and other spp. of Cola.
Coriander	Coriandrum sativum L.
Cumin (cummin)	Cuminum cyminum L.
Curacao orange peel (orange, bitter peel)	Citrus aurantium L.
Cusparia bark	Galipea officinalis Hancock.
Dandelion	Taraxacum officinale Weber and T. laevigatum DC.

Dandelion root	Do.
Dog grass (quackgrass, triticum)	Agropyron repens (L.) Beauv.
Elder flowers	Sambucus canadensis L. and S. nigra I.
Estragole (esdragol, esdragon, tarragon)	Artemisia dracunculus L.
Estragon (tarragon)	Do.
Fennel, sweet	Foeniculum vulgare Mill.
Fenugreek	Trigonella foenum-graecum L.
Galanga (galangal)	Alpinia officinarum Hance.
Geranium	Pelargonium spp.
Geranium, East Indian	Cymbopogon martini Stapf.
Geranium, rose	Pelargonium graveolens L'Her.
Ginger	Zingiber officinale Rosc.
Grapefruit	Citrus paradisi Macf.
Guava	Psidium spp.
Hickory bark	Carya spp.
Horehound (hoarhound)	Marrubium vulgare L.
Hops	Humulus lupulus L.
Horsemint	Monarda punctata L.
Hyssop	Hyssopus officinalis L.
Immortelle	Helichrysum augustifolium DC.
Jasmine	Jasminum officinale L. and other spp. of Jasminum.
Juniper (berries)	Juniperus communis L.
Kola nut	Cola acuminata Schott and Endl., and other spp. of Cola.
Laurel berries	Laurus nobilis L.
Laurel leaves	Laurus spp.
Lavender	Lavandula officinalis Chaix.
Lavender, spike	Lavandula latifolia Vill.
Lavandin	Hybrids between Lavandula officinalis Chaix and Lavandula latifolin Vill.
Lemon	Citrus limon (L.) Burm. f.
Lemon balm (see balm)	
Lemon grass	Cymbopogon citratus DC. and Cymbopogon lexuosus Stapf.
Lemon peel	Citrus limon (L.) Burm. f.
Lime	Citrus aurantifolia Swingle.
Linden flowers	Tilia spp.
Locust bean	Ceratonia siliqua L,
Lupulin	Humulus lupulus L.
Mace	Myristica fragrans Houtt.
Mandarin	Citrus reticulata Blanco.
Marjoram, sweet	Majorana hortensis Moench.
Mate	Ilex paraguariensis St. Hil.
Melissa (see balm)	
Menthol	Mentha spp.
Menthyl acetate	Do.
Molasses (extract)	Saccarum officinarum L.
Mustard	Brassica spp.
Naringin	Citrus paradisi Macf.
Neroli, bigarade	Citrus aurantium L.
Nutmeg	Myristica fragrans Houtt.

Onion	Allium cepa L.
Orange, bitter, flowers	Citrus aurantium L.
Orange, bitter, peel	Do.
Orange leaf	Citrus sinensis (L.) Osbeck.
Orange, sweet	Do.
Orange, sweet, flowers	Do.
Orange, sweet, peel	Do.
Origanum	Origanum spp.
Palmarosa	Cymbopogon martini Stapf.
Paprika	Capsicum annuum L.
Parsley	Petroselinum crispum (Mill.) Mansf.
Pepper, black	Piper nigrum L.
Pepper, white	Do.
Peppermint	Mentha piperita L.
Peruvian balsam	Myroxylon pereirae Klotzsch.
Petitgrain	Citrus aurantium L.
Petitgrain lemon	Citrus limon (L.) Burm. f.
Petitgrain mandarin or tangerine	Citrus reticulata Blanco.
Pimenta	Pimenta officinalis Lindl.
Pimenta leaf	Pimenta officinalis Lindl.
Pipsissewa leaves	Chimaphila umbellata Nutt.
Pomegranate	Punica granatum L.
Prickly ash bark	Xanthoxylum (or Zanthoxylum) Americanum Mill. or Xanthoxylum clava-herculis L.
Rose absolute	Rosa alba L., Rosa centifolia L., Rosa damascena Mill., Rosa gallica L., and vars. of spp.
Rose (otto of roses, attar of roses)	Do.
Rose buds	Do.
Rose flowers	Do.
Rose fruit (hips)	Do.
Rose geranium	Pelargonium graveolens L'Her.
Rose leaves	Rosa spp.
Rosemary	Rosmarinus officinalis L.
Saffron	Crocus sativus L.
Sage	Salvia officinalis L.
Sage, Greek	Salvia triloba L.
Sage, Spanish	Salvia lavandulaefolia Vahl.
St. John's bread	Ceratonia siliqua L.
Savory, summer	Satureia hortensis L.
Savory, winter	Satureia montana L.
Schinus molle	Schinus molle L.
Sloe berries (blackthorn berries)	Prunus spinosa L.
Spearmint	Mentha spicata L.
Spike lavender	Lavandula latifolia Vill.
Tamarind	Tamarindus indica L.
Tangerine	Citrus reticulata Blanco.
Tarragon	Artemisia dracunculus L.
Tea	Thea sinensis L.
Thyme	Thymus vulgaris L. and Thymus zygis var. gracilis Boiss.

Thyme, white	Do.
Thyme, wild or creeping	Thymus serpyllum L.
Triticum (see dog grass)	
Tuberose	Polianthes tuberosa L.
Turmeric	Curcuma longa L.
Vanilla	Vanilla planifolia Andr. or Vanilla tahitensis J. W. Moore.
Violet flowers	Viola odorata L.
Violet leaves	Do.
Violet leaves absolute	Do.
Wild cherry bark	Prunus serotina Ehrh.
Ylang-ylang	Cananga odorata Hook. f. and Thoms.
Zedoary bark	Curcuma zedoaria Rosc.

www.ingramcontent.com/pod-product-compliance
Lightning Source LLC
Chambersburg PA
CBHW081121280526
45787CB00007B/2928